I0455143

Miracles Do Happen!

KRYSTLE J. LYNCH

Copyright © 2012 Krystle Lynch

Editing by: Elizabeth Bellinger

Disclaimer: This book is not intended as a substitute for the medical advice of physicians. The reader should regularly consult a physician in matters relating to his/her health and particularly with respect to any symptoms that may require diagnosis or medical attention.

All rights reserved.

ISBN-10: 1479111775
ISBN-13: 978-1479111770

www.krystlelynch.wix.com/author

DEDICATION

This book is dedicated first and foremost to my **Lord and savior Jesus Christ**. Thank You for bringing me through every trial, and giving me two beautiful children and one on the way.

To my husband **Gabriel**: I love you, and thank you for believing in me every step of the way. You always push me to the next level.

To my Children **Gabe III** and **Kingston**: I am so blessed to have children such as you. Every day that I look at you I am reminded of how much prayer it took to get you here. I love you, and let this book be a keepsake for you to know what God has done.

*In loving memory of our baby girl Sarah.

KRYSTLE LYNCH

Special Thanks to: Janet Depass (my mother), **Patrick Depass** (my father), **Gabriel Sr.** and **Viana Lynch** (my husband's parents), **Keisha Hurlock** and **Hunter Depass** (my sister and brother), **Nate Lynch** and **Jemina Lynch** (my husband's brother and sister), **Julie Calderon** (my aunt), **Donna Brown** (my aunt), **Tamika Riley** (my cousin), **Gloria Brown** (my grandmother), **Pastor Riva Tims**, **Apostle Andre Williams** and **Pastor Jocelyn Williams** (my pastors). All of you played a very important role in the stories of these miracles.

CONTENTS

INTRODUCTION

It is my prayer that as you read my story, you will be strengthened. I pray that the Holy Spirit will heal every part of you that is hurting. Know that God is always with you and sees every hurt.

God is still performing miracles today. Maybe the doctor has told you that you cannot have children, Gods word says that you can. Maybe you've had multiple miscarriages. Maybe you have had difficult pregnancies, Gods word says that you are healed.

I pray that every woman that reads this book will be renewed and encouraged. God is no respecter of persons, and will do just what he said he would do.

Chapter 1

GOD IS MY STRENGTH

It was the spring of May 2004 that my husband and I got married. As husband and wife, and even while dating, we talked about the future. How many children we wanted was at the top of the list. I wanted two, while my husband wanted four. Then in October of 2004 our Pastor at the time gave us a prophetic word that said we were going to conceive a child soon. People around me started asking if I was pregnant, which I wasn't at that time; but a few months later in February of 2005, we were pregnant. Excitement wasn't a big enough word to explain how we felt; we were overjoyed, and elated! Things were going great. I had just started a temp job as a teacher and was thankful for the opportunity. Our family was so happy.

I went to all my scheduled doctor's appointments. We told our parents that we were pregnant around 8 weeks. The rest of our extended families found out at around 10 weeks. I remember talking to my Aunt about Ob Gyn's that she knew of. One thing she said was that the doctor wouldn't see me until about 12 weeks. I was so anxious to see what was going on inside of me. The first appointment was the normal routine. Though there was a lot of paper work to fill out with our family history, hearing my baby's heart beat for the first time was amazing!

At around 12 weeks, I was having some bleeding, and the doctor restricted me from doing certain things. That summer I didn't have a job so I started sending out my resume. I got an interview with the exact school that I wanted to work for. When I got a call and I got the job I was so excited. Accepting this job would mean that I would be a full time teacher. The job was offered to me in May, but I didn't start until August.

Summer ended and August was here; school was about to start. The week before school, there was a new teachers orientation and I had to do a lot of walking. My classroom was in a portable, way in the back of the school. During the first week of school, I was able to meet my students and finish decorating my classroom. The first week of school finished so quickly; the next thing I knew it was Saturday.

That Saturday in August, I was home by myself. My Husband went to work, but something just wasn't right. My stomach was hurting, but this wasn't just any ordinary stomach ache. I called my husband and tried to explain to him what was happening. He thought maybe

I just need to drink some water and sit down. We didn't know what to expect. I called my mother and Aunt who are nurses and they said go to the hospital. I called my husband back again and he came. On the way to the hospital the pain was getting more intense, so much that I started to moan. Early labor was far from my mind, because I had never experienced child birth before. There I lay in the back seat of the car, praying to get to the hospital fast.

We finally arrived at the nearest hospital. When we arrived I was hooked up to all kinds of machines to monitor contractions. The doctors tried to give me medication to stop the contractions, but my heart rate was too high. There was nothing that could be done. We put all of our trust in God. My husband called everyone he knew that would intercede for our unborn baby, because it was too early for him to be born.

My Ob finally arrived, and he got there in the nick of time. It was then time to push. I couldn't believe what was happening. I didn't know what it meant to have a baby this early. I was given an episiotomy to protect our baby's fragile body. A few minutes later, Gabriel III was born. He was suctioned and intubated by the best neonatologist in town. The Neonatologist wasn't scheduled to be at this hospital when I arrived. God allowed him to be at the right place at the right time.

Neonatology is a subspecialty of pediatrics that consists of the medical care of newborn infants, especially the ill or premature newborn infant. It is a hospital-based specialty, and is usually practiced in neonatal intensive care units (NICUs). The principal patients of neonatologists are newborn infants who are ill or requiring special medical care due to prematurity, low birth weight, intrauterine growth retardation, congenital malformations (birth defects), sepsis, or birth asphyxias.

I finally got to see him before he was transferred to another hospital. There he was, Gabe, alive and fighting at only 1 pound 8 ounces. At 24 weeks gestation he was considered a premature baby. As he was moving all around in the incubator; I looked at him in shock. I still didn't understand what had happened. My husband, Mom and Aunt were there. My Aunt said, touch his hand. As I touched his hand I couldn't believe what I was seeing. I had never seen a premature baby before, and didn't know what to expect.

While all of this was going on, we were supposed to be closing on the sale of our house. We had to postpone the closing due to Gabriel's early birth. The buyers were gracious enough to allow us to do this until I got out of the hospital.

Gabriel and I were also being transferred to a different hospital, and after we got there, we were able to see Gabe in the **Neonatal intensive care unit** (NICU). The (NICU) is

an intensive care unit specializing in the
care of ill or premature newborn infants.
He looked so fragile, and could fit in the
palm of my hand. Gabriel had several
nasogastric (NG) tubes. An NG tube is
a small thin tube that ran through his
nose into his stomach, so he could eat.
There were also tubes in his throat to
help him breath. The Doctors told us
that he would be in the Nicu for a very
long time. I asked, "What's a long
time?". They said it depended on how
he did, but that the minimum was three
months.

I cried almost every day, until our
baby came home. It was hard to see my
one pound baby getting poked and
prodded by needles and IV's. Wherever
there was a vein, that's where an IV
went. He even had an IV in his
forehead. There were many types of
medicines that were given to him, one
was for reflux. When we took him
home, he had severe reflux and would
throw up half of his bottle. One of the

medications he took for reflux was reglan. Even with this medicine, he still had severe reflux. It was to the point that he had to sit in his car seat for about an hour with no movement, to digest his food. I know they say that babies don't remember their pain but as a first time mother I felt his pain. Gabriel's weight gain was always something we were concerned about. The pediatrician put him on Neosure, a formula for premature babies. This formula had extra nutrients and calories that assisted with his weight gain.

After about six weeks in the hospital we were alerted that Gabe had *Patent ductus arteriosus* (**PDA**) and would need a (PDA) ligation. A (PDA) ligation is a condition in which the ductus arteriosus does not close. The word "patent" means open. The ductus arteriosus is a blood vessel that allows blood to go around the baby's lungs before birth. Soon after the infant is born and the lungs fill with air, the ductus arteriosus is no longer needed. It usually closes in a couple of days after birth. Having an open ductus arteriosus, leads to abnormal blood flow between the aorta and pulmonary artery, (two major blood vessels that carry blood from the heart).

We went back and forth with the doctors trying to decide where to have his surgery. One of the local hospitals offered it. The hospital Gabriel was at wanted to fly him to Tampa by helicopter. We were concerned that Gabriel's fragile body would be affected during the flight. The doctors insured us that he would be fine and wanted to keep the surgery within their system. We finally agreed. I can remember the flight team preparing him to go into the helicopter. As they flew, we drove. Gabriel's surgery took approximately ten minutes.

Gabriel also had Retinopathy of prematurity (ROP). (ROP) is a disease that primarily occurs in premature babies. It causes abnormal blood vessels to grow in the retina, the layer of nerve tissue in the eye that enables us to see. This growth can cause the retina to detach from the back of the eye, leading to blindness.

In Gabe's case he had this surgery. Going to the NICU almost every day was something I would have to prepare myself for. Every night and day for three months we would visit. Our gas bill was astronomical. There were many nights of eating out, so that we could spend time with our son. During the days my Aunt would pick me up and take me to the hospital. I would see some very sick infants and others that were doing ok. Some parents didn't know if tomorrow their child would still be alive. It was hard to see my child and others, hurting. Tears flooded my eyes almost every time that I stepped into the Nicu.

Throughout the first couple of weeks, I was asked to pump for breast milk. I got some at first, but I just couldn't get any more out. Breast milk can be vital for premature babies, to help their immune system. I just couldn't produce. I was offered the breast milk of other mothers, which is sterilized. We declined; I couldn't stomach the fact that my child would be getting another mother's milk. I felt as if I had failed. My child laying there fighting for his life, and I can't give him my milk.

I "Kangaroo cared" as much as possible, to make sure that my baby would know his mother. Kangaroo care is the practice of holding your diapered baby on your bare chest (if you're the father) or between your breasts (if you're the mother), with a blanket draped over your baby's back. Kangaroo care helps your premature baby gain weight, regulate the heart and breathing, and has many other benefits. A few years ago there was a story about a premature baby that died after delivery at 27 weeks. The mother kangaroo cared for two hours, and miraculously the baby woke up. Doctors were amazed!

Each day he grew stronger. As Gabe grew, he would take the nasal canula out of his nose and pull the I'Vs out of his arm. We would get weekly updates on his status. One week they told us that he had a grade 4 bleed, then the next week they told us that he had cerebral palsy. The next week something else. Imagine how stressful that was. Gabe was finally released at five pounds. He was sent home with an apnea monitor, just in case he choked or stopped breathing.

There were many elderly volunteers that made Gabriel tons of crocheted preemie hats and blankets, for us to take home. My youngest sister in law Jemina made some also. Gabriel's preemie clothes and diapers were so small, you would think they were for a baby doll. The only way we could make it was with God and the prayers of others. In situations like these family support is critical. At that time we were offered help from our church. The church offered to make cooked meals, and we also received help from family, and friends. The hospital also provided a lot of support from counseling to premature baby education. We were covered on ever side. If you are in a similar situation right now, know that God is there with you. The church can be a great support, and many churches offer free counseling.

God will give you strength and comfort. It is ok to cry and God will wipe away every tear. Others may not understand your pain, but God is a comforter and healer. God can work in any situation. No matter what the doctors say. GOD HAS THE FINAL SAY SO!

"The scripture states in Luke chapter 1: 6-25 .
And they were both righteous before God, walking in all the commandments and ordinances of the Lord blameless. And they had no child, because that Elisabeth was barren, and they both were now well stricken in years. And it came to pass, that while he executed the priest's office before God in the order of his course,

According to the custom of the priest's office, his lot was
to burn incense when he went into the temple of the Lord.
And the whole multitude of the people were
praying without at the time of incense. And there
appeared unto him an angel of the Lord standing on the
right side of the altar of incense. And when Zacharias saw
him, he was troubled, and fear fell upon him. But the
angel said unto him, Fear not, Zacharias: for thy prayer is
heard; and thy wife Elisabeth shall bear thee a son,
and thou shalt call his name John. And thou shalt have joy
and gladness; and many shall rejoice at his birth. For he
shall be great in the sight of the Lord, and shall
drink neither wine nor strong drink; and he shall be filled
with the Holy Ghost, even from his mother's womb. And
many of the children of Israel shall he turn to
the Lord their God. And he shall go before him in the
spirit and power of Elias, to turn the hearts of the fathers
to the children, and the disobedient to the wisdom of
the just; to make ready a people prepared for the Lord.
And Zacharias said unto the angel, Whereby shall I know
this? for I am an old man, and my wife well stricken
in years. And the angel answering said unto him, I am
Gabriel, that stand in the presence of God; and am sent to
speak unto thee, and to shew thee these glad tidings. And,
behold, thou shalt be dumb, and not able to speak, until
the day that these things shall be performed, because thou
believest not my words, which shall be fulfilled in their
season. And the people waited for Zacharias, and marveled
that he tarried so long in the temple. And when he came
out, he could not speak unto them: and they perceived that
he had seen a vision in the temple: for he beckoned unto
them, and remained speechless. And it came to pass, that,
as soon as the days of his ministration were accomplished,
he departed to his own house. And after those days his
wife Elisabeth conceived, and hid herself five months,
saying, Thus hath the Lord dealt with me in the days

wherein he looked on me, to take away my reproach among men. "

Zacharias asked God for a son. In those days, he could have put his wife Elizabeth away for not being able to give him a child. God heard his cry while he was in the temple. Both he and his wife were well over age to have a child, but the angel Gabriel reassured him and even told him of his child's destiny. Zachariah couldn't speak until his child was born, because he didn't believe. Elizabeth conceived John (the Baptist) and hid her pregnancy for 5 months. Many that have gone through miscarrying will not share their pregnancy until they are over the three month mark. I have done this myself. Just as Elizabeth conceived a miracle, your child can be a miracle also… just believe! I know believing can be hard sometimes, because it takes action. But if God did it for me, he can do it for you!

Prayer for your baby:

God, this child is here for a reason. There is a plan, purpose and destiny for this baby. I pray for a full recovery in Jesus name. I speak life to my premature baby that is in the hospital now or just now coming home. Every negative doctors report is turning around for the good in Jesus name. This child will not have any difficulties in life and will play, talk and walk like other children. Thank you Lord for touching the hand of every doctor, they will call this child a miracle baby. Amen.

Chapter 2

THE NEGATIVE AND POSITIVE

Throughout the whole process, people either responded negatively or positively to my situation. My husband and I had the support of our families, which I thank God for. I especially remember my grandmother making my favorite soup, Turkey soup with lots of beans. I had leftovers for weeks. My mother Janet would play soothing Christian music while Gabe slept in the hospital and she would also bring us cooked meals. When Gabe had his surgery, my mother in law Viana brought a family friend whose child had just also went through a trying time. This gave us encouragement, letting us know that God is in control. They checked on us constantly and visited Gabe weekly. The staff in the NICU was the best. They made us feel confident about the care Gabriel was getting. We also received phone calls from others that went through the same thing.

On the other hand, sometimes people who have never been through these types of situations will say things and not realize what they just said. People said things like, look at so and so, they are in a worse situation, you need to get over it and stop crying. Sometimes, I would think to myself, "did they really just say that?" Thank God that the good overrides the bad.

I still had the question in the back of my mind. What did I do to deserve this? I would look around at others having full term babies. This made me feel sad, in a way, because I didn't get to take my baby home the same day. My baby shower was while Gabriel was in the hospital, and it was beautiful. My whole family really made sure that I didn't miss out. My sister Keisha flew all the way from Ohio. Everyone made sure we had what we needed. Although this was still a tough time, I knew that God would not let me down. I kept asking God, "Why?" God said, I will not put on you more than you can bare. The devil may have thought that he was going to take our child, but when God has a purpose and destiny locked up in that child, there is nothing the devil can do to stop it. God will always fulfill his promises!

After 4 weeks I went back to work as a teacher. Working kept my mind off of my child being in the hospital. It was still tough though. I remember crying in front of the students one day, because I just couldn't take it anymore. The students said "What's wrong Mrs. Lynch?". I had to quickly wipe my tears away and proceed with class. I responded to my students as if my eyes were just watery.

Everyone at the school was so supportive; both teachers and administration. I received phone calls from a lot of teachers and the administration and to this day they still remember me because of this situation. Finally in November of 2005, it was time for Gabriel to come home. My husband and I decided that I would stay home with him, because of the intense care that he would need. Since the teachers and staff weren't able to throw me a baby shower, they sent me lots of baby gifts. I was so grateful for all that was done for us.

We had doctor's visits every week. There were several different specialist we went to, including, ophthalmology, pulmonologist, cardiology, ENT, pediatrician, and the developmental specialist. This continued for the first year. Every year after, the appointments became less. Gabriel progressed and his pediatrician was proud of his results. Now Gabriel only visits those specialist once per year, and the pulmonologist every three to six months. Currently our first son is a healthy and happy seven year old. He has no medical problems, and he is our Miracle child. To God be the glory!

Chapter 3

THE UNEXPECTED

This pregnancy had started the same as usual. Since I had a premature delivery in the last pregnancy; the doctors told me that I would need a cerclage. A cerclage is a surgical stitch used for an incompetent cervix. I was seeing all types of doctors; this included high risk Doctors to really make sure that this pregnancy was successful. I was having a lot of pain from a pinched nerve that didn't seem to go away with my first son. My blood work had come back and my HCG levels were high. The Doctors asked if twins run in either side of our family. An ultrasound was performed to see what was going on inside my womb but there was only one baby.

When they did an ultrasound, they found a large cyst, and this was the cause of my pain. It was around 14 weeks that a cerclage was suggested to me. My husband and I felt as if we were being forced into getting this procedure. The more the doctors pushed, the more we didn't want the procedure.

On the day of the elections, in November 2008, at about 16 weeks pregnant, I was sitting at home and my water broke. I called my husband, and he rushed home. I called the doctor, and he said just keep your legs up. I laid on my back on a sheet in the back of my husband's van with my legs up, trying to get the water to stop leaking. The water was gushing out. We arrived at the hospital. I was in a wheel chair being rolled to the maternity unit. As we got to the unit. I explained the situation. The person I spoke with looked at me and said there is probably nothing they can do. My heart sank. I said to myself, "God you are a God of miracles you did it for us before, and you can do it again".

There is a term called Fetal viability (Roe vs. Wade case 1973), this law puts a limit on care given if a baby was born severely premature. I didn't know that this existed, and found this out during this pregnancy. Our 24 weeker had just made it. In the past, before all of the advanced technology, fetal viability was only 28 weeks. Now it is 24 weeks. From 23 weeks or less doctors have the right to refuse to treat a baby, unless the parent insist. And even then, a doctor can still refuse. Doctors fear that saving a baby that is 23 weeks will be more harm than good. It has been documented that these babies have more chance of a disability, and a harder time in life. Every state is different but I believe that it should be up to the parents to decide.

I was taken to a room on the unit, and had many ultrasounds, even repeated ultrasounds to see if a miracle had occurred. The doctor called by phone and said, "we are going to have to terminate this pregnancy". He said there is no more amniotic fluid around the baby, and if we wait any longer you can get an infection which will make things worse. There was nothing that could be done. I cried out to God and asked " why?" This child was prophesied. "How can your word not come to pass?" What I had just experienced was a miscarriage. A miscarriage is the naturally occurring expulsion of a nonviable fetus and placenta from the uterus; also known as spontaneous abortion or pregnancy loss.

It was time to deliver and at that time we didn't find out what the gender of the baby was yet. I was given tablets to make me go into labor. After a few minutes, the baby was out. There was a lot of blood loss. The nurses took the baby and cleaned the body off. After they cleaned the baby, I asked what the gender was. They said, it is a girl. Our angel Sarah was brought to me in a small basket, fully formed with all her limbs. I couldn't believe what I was seeing. So many things went through my mind. I said, "God, what have I done to deserve this? I have followed you and served you, and seen others who have done things to lose their child; and still have healthy pregnancies. I don't get it!" At that point, I realized that some things have no explanation, and we don't know why God allows things to happen the way they do. All I know is that God, the creator of heaven and earth is in control.

I thank God for my husband, mother, father, and family that supported us during this time. Having a support system can help you in your recovery from grief. If you don't have family support, the hospital has many resources. After all of this, we were given the option to have a funeral or allow the hospital to bury the baby at a disclosed location. We chose for the hospital to take care of it. The hospital took pictures of our little girl, for us to take home. Every time I looked at them I would cry. We will never forget her; she will always be in our heart. A young teen volunteer at the hospital made us a memoir in which her foot prints are on. To this day her footprints are still on my dresser.

The next day it was time for me to get up and about. I had lost so much blood, I was feeling faint; and I was afraid to get up. I asked the nursing staff if I could just use the bed pan to use the bathroom, but they insisted that I go to the restroom. I got to the toilet ok, but after I sat down, I looked at the nurse and said I feel nauseous. The next thing you know my eyes rolled to the back of my head, and I was on the floor. My mother was frantic. My husband called for help from the other nurses on the floor. The nurse put something under my nose that would make me wake up. I finally woke up. After I woke up, all I remember was my mother saying; "pick her up now", and put her on the bed. My mother is also a nurse and she knew what lots of blood loss meant, but nobody knew how much blood I had lost. After this ordeal, my blood count was checked, and it dropped all the way to seven.

While at the hospital, I received a lot of phone calls from friends and family. It was surprising to hear some of them tell me their stories of miscarriage and loss. I knew then that I wasn't alone. Some people said they were sorry to hear what happened, and others didn't say anything at all. Then there were some that made negative comments. A lot of times people can be very insensitive. I chose to… ignore the comments and still love them. People will always assume that they know how you feel; when they have no idea. God is the only one that can truly see your hurt.

Prayer for peace during a loss:

Father God I ask you for peace during this time. It is so difficult to see past losing our unborn child. Send your Holy Spirit to comfort me. I know that joy cometh in the morning. Restore what has been lost. I trust your plan and purpose for my life, and I put everything in your hands.

Chapter 4

SPIRITUAL WARFARE

It was finally time for me to go home. Going home without my little girl was hard. I needed the peace of God to be with me. When I came home, I was still grieving for our lost child. I thought that I was ok, but then I started to have anxiety attacks, and many sleepless nights. I would pray and they would get worse. I remember one Sunday while at church, I broke down in tears. One of the ministers came up to me and embraced me. Although she had never been through what I had, she said you know the word of God, so this is not a faith thing. At that point realized that this was a spiritual attack. You see, the enemy will attack when he thinks your vulnerable and at your weakest state. The enemy wants you to stop praying and go into a depressive state, but you have to keep praying and pressing.

Here are some tactics that the enemy tried to use against me when going through with my first birth, and the loss of our second child. The tactics were fatigue, fear, feeling forsaken, and blaming myself. The enemy will try to wear you out spiritually to the point of giving up on having any more children. I combated this by prayer and fasting. It seemed like I was on a fast every day for at least three months. The things that I was experiencing, I couldn't talk to everyone about. I had to shut everything out except the Lord's voice. He began to speak and I was given a vision of the enemies plan. The enemy also wants to attack with the spirit of fear. I began to wonder if I would ever have a full term child. I didn't understand why I was having difficult pregnancies. The enemy will flood your mind with thoughts that God has forsaken you and forgotten about you. Know that God has not forgotten about you. God will never leave you nor forsake you (Deuteronomy 31:6). The enemy will make it seem as if what happened was your fault. You may have replayed the events that lead up to your loss or preterm birth. We cannot control how our bodies respond in pregnancy, but with prayer we can call those things that be not as though they were.

Miscarriage and preterm birth happen for many different reasons. No matter what the reason, God is still in control. God can heal your body from the inside out. The enemy's tactics must be rebuked in Jesus name. If you have had multiple miscarriages you must pray against curses spoken over you or your family line. There may be a generational curse that needs to be broken. You must also rebuke bareness. Exodus 23:26

states that "There shall nothing miscarry, nor be barren, in your land: the number of your days I will fulfill". This powerful scripture can be a reality for you. This is a scripture that you can confess on a daily basis. Confess that there will be no miscarriage or barrenness in your land. With Prayer and Praise the devil has to flee. I continued to put the word into action, and the attacks ceased. Thank God for the blood of Jesus.

Spiritual warfare prayer:

I break every curse spoken over me by others in Jesus name. Every generational curse stemming back to my forefathers is broken in Jesus name. I am fruitful and my seed will multiply in the earth. I come against barrenness, miscarriage, preterm labor and preterm birth in Jesus name. I cast down the spirit of fear and pull down every stronghold in Jesus name.

Chapter 5

THE MAKING OF A KING

"Oh my" I replied. "There are two lines". My husband replied "Are you serious?" I took two or three test, and it was the same result. I put everything in God's hands and said, "Lord you know all things, have your way". I thought, "How is this pregnancy going to turn out. Every child that I conceive, I dedicate to the Lord while they are in the womb. There is nothing like when a mother dedicates her child, just like Hannah did.

"Samuel 1:9-25 states, Once when they had finished eating and drinking in Shiloh, Hannah stood up. Now Eli the priest was sitting on his chair by the doorpost of the LORD's house. In her deep anguish Hannah prayed to the LORD, weeping bitterly. And she made a

vow, saying, "LORD Almighty , if you will only look on your servant's misery and remember me, and not forget your servant but give her a son, then I will give him to the LORD for all the days of his life, and no razor will ever be used on his head." As she kept on praying to the LORD, Eli observed her mouth. Hannah was praying in her heart, and her lips were moving but her voice was not heard. Eli thought she was drunk and said to her, "How long are you going to stay drunk? Put away your wine." "Not so, my lord," Hannah replied, "I am a woman who is deeply troubled. I have not been drinking wine or beer; I was pouring out my soul to the LORD. Do not take your servant for a wicked woman; I have been praying here out of my great anguish and grief." Eli answered, "Go in peace, and may the God of Israel grant you what you have asked of him. "She said, "May your servant find favor in your eyes. " Then she went her way and ate something, and her face was no longer downcast. Early the next morning they arose and worshiped before the LORD and then went back to their home at Ramah. Elkanah made love to his wife Hannah, and
the LORD remembered her. So in the course of time Hannah became pregnant and gave birth to a son. She named him Samuel, saying, "Because I asked the LORD for him." When her husband Elkanah went up with all his family to offer the annual sacrifice to the LORD and to fulfill his vow, Hannah did not go. She said to her husband, "After the boy is weaned, I will take him and present him before the LORD, and he will live there always." "Do what seems best to you," her husband Elkanah told her. "Stay here until you have weaned him; only may the LORD make good his word." So the woman stayed at home and nursed her son until she had weaned him. After he was weaned, she took the boy with her, young as he was, along with a three-year-old bull, an ephah of flour and a skin of wine, and brought him to the house of the LORD at Shiloh. When the bull

had been sacrificed, they brought the boy to Eli, and she said to him, "Pardon me, my lord. As surely as you live, I am the woman who stood here beside you praying to the LORD. I prayed for this child, and the LORD has granted me what I asked of him. So now I give him to the LORD. For his whole life he will be given over to the LORD." And he worshiped the LORD there."

Hannah promised the Lord that if He would give her a son, that she would dedicate him to the Lord. Instead of allowing others to make her bitter, she began to pray. Prayer and faith are what I believe moved God to work on her behalf. Miracles can come forth through prayer. Samuel was birthed out of prayer.

At 10 weeks pregnant, I scheduled a regular first time Ob appointment. This was the first time that I had been to this doctor. The doctor reviewed my records and history and this is where the negativity began. As my husband and I sat in the office, the doctor began to pull apart my pregnancy history. He began by saying you delivered your first child at 24 weeks and lost your second. It doesn't look good for this pregnancy.

I stated. "What would make you say that?". The Doctor replied; "I don't think that you're going to carry this child past X amount of weeks, due to your history". He was very nonchalant, and had no interest in helping me carry my baby to term. I thought, what kind of Doctor would tell you good luck with this pregnancy? If I hadn't been through what I had been through in the past I would have cried. Something in me rose up and said no, this is not God's will. I came against everything that doctor said with the word of God and spoke to my womb. I told my husband, I need to change doctors.

The first thing I did was call my Aunt. She works in the Ob field and knows a lot of great doctors. She referred me to a different one, and from that point on my experience was wonderful. My Aunt called and made the first appointment for me. Without her help, it could have taken a month or so just to get an appointment. She also told the Doctor that I needed a cerclage asap. By the next week, I was in my new OB's office and had an appointment with a High Risk doctor the week after . Everything happened so quickly. After my High Risk appointment, the Doctor says we are going to schedule your cerclage for Friday, which was only 4 days away. It is normal to be nervous, and I was. I thought oh my goodness, but I knew I had to do this procedure for my baby. So at 13 weeks, I was being prepped for surgery.

I read about cerclages online. Reading was my only way to see what others experienced and also the success rates. They say the earlier you have the procedure the better and there's less risk. After being prepped, the baby's heart rate is checked, then the Doctor visits you. You are then visited by the anesthesiologist. Next, you are rolled into the operating room. An epidural is placed so that you are numb waist down. Once you are numb the procedure begins. A special instrument is used to open the vaginal canal, and your cervix is stitched tight. After the procedure, there is bleeding, but very minimal. You are rolled back to the recovery room, and the baby's heart rate is checked again. Recovery takes about four hours, time for the anesthesia to wear off and to check the status of your bleeding. In my case everything went great and I went home the same day.

When you get home you will need help for about a week. You must limit walking and household duties to make sure that you heal properly. After the week you can ease into going back to your regular schedule. Every woman is different; some women can go back to work with a Cerclage and others may have to be on bed rest. In my case, I was on partial bed rest. I could go to church and then sit down; go to the grocery store to maybe get one item, but with very limited walking. Although I had a cerclage placed, I still took many precautions. Some would say, why don't you go here, or there? My husband and I discussed it and we felt that if I needed to lay out on the couch every day for this baby to get here; then that's what I would do. At the end of the day, when people make comments, they are not the ones that will have to care for this child, if the child was born too early. It would be the responsibility of my husband and I.

The weeks went by and everything was looking good. It was time to find out the sex of the baby. My husband didn't want to know this time. I was so eager to know, that we found out anyway. The Ultrasound tech said "It's A Boy". I said check it again. The tech said, "It's still a boy". Since I went to the High Risk Doctor every other week, I was able to double check and verify the gender. We were excited to have another boy, and Gabe would have someone to play with. We had a few names in mind, and decided to name him Kingston.

At around 22 weeks, I began contracting. I went to the OR (operating room) because the contractions wouldn't stop. The doctor then put me on Procardia, to help with the contractions and blood pressure simultaneously. Once on these medications the contractions ceased and my blood pressure was better than ever before. I was blessed again to get the help of my mother and mother in law with household duties. My mother and aunt came one weekend and cleaned and de-cluttered our house from top to bottom. My mother in law came every week to bring us dinner, a couple of days in a row.

Passing the 24 week mark was a milestone for me. So I had my own little celebration with each week that passed. The next thing you know, I was 33 weeks pregnant. I thought, Wow, I have never experienced pregnancy at this stage. The contractions started again, even while taking the medicine. I called the doctor and the first thing that he said was, it's Braxton Hicks. So I started to time my contractions. He then raised the medication to a higher dose. After monitoring the contractions for about three days I said something isn't right; these contractions are not going away.

I went to the ER, and was monitored by a machine for contractions. I was monitored for a few hours and then sent home. Two days later, while at home, the contractions started again. At the time, I would go to the doctor's office to be monitored by a machine once per week. During this pregnancy I had several UTI's(urinary tract infection), and while all these contractions were going on the doctor put me on an antibiotic. He gave me a stronger antibiotic than before to kill the bacteria, but I was allergic to the antibiotic and my heart rate went into the 140s-150s while at rest. I went back to the ER and the doctor's couldn't figure out why my body was reacting this way since the last time I took the medicine was a day ago. I was also feverish, and just didn't feel right. The doctor's said we are going to keep you over night so that we can find out what is going on.

I was sent for an x-ray to check my lungs and heart for blood clots. Thankfully everything was normal. The contraction machine was hooked back up and I was being sent to the cardiac unit. I stayed on this unit for one week. The cardiologist visited me every day and I was given multiple tests to check my heart, but my heart was fine. My heart rate went back up into the 120's. The cardiac unit could not release me until my heart rate was within safe limits. Since everything was ok, it was time for me to go back to the labor and delivery unit. I also stayed on this unit for one week. My husband and son would stay with me almost every night.

The next week, the contractions were getting worse, and I was 35 weeks pregnant. Magnesium Sulfate was placed through my IV to help with the contractions; this was one of the most horrible experiences in my whole entire life. One minute I was hot, one minute cold, and my head was spinning. I just wanted to be off of this medicine, the nurses said this will help to stop preterm labor. Finally the contractions slowed down and then a day later started up again.

They started to monitor the baby's heart rate even more, and it kept dropping periodically. I was 35 weeks and 6 days, and the baby's heart rate was dropping too much and an emergency C-section was scheduled. Kingston was born and the cord was wrapped around his neck, and that's why his heart rate kept dropping. Thank God that I didn't deliver vaginally. God always has a way of working everything out. Finally my Precious Kingston was here, at five pounds eight ounces and I made it to almost full term. Glory be to God, He gave us another miracle baby.

God's word will not turn back to you void. That which He said He would do will come to past. There were many oppositions, especially early on during this pregnancy, but my faith in God kept me going. I was determined to deliver this baby. God is a miracle working God. God anointed the hands of every doctor and nurse that tended to me. I believe God has placed knowledge and expertise in earthly doctors for a reason. Because of the invention of the Cerclage, I am able to carry the rest of my babies to term.

There is a spiritual and natural element here. Spiritually we must speak the word of God, and believe His word. Naturally, we must do everything humanly possible to help our situation. This means, going to the doctor to get checkups, getting my cerclage, and being monitored more closely. I will never know what would have happened if I would have gotten a cerclage with the baby I lost. My belief is that I would have carried longer. I have heard many stories in which people said that they were believing God to heal them. I strongly believe that God can do the impossible, but we must do our part.

God still does supernatural miracles, and then there are those that have to take medicine for their condition or need to have surgery. God wouldn't have created these professionals for no reason. Now, if God tells you that He is going to heal you and that you don't need any medical help, then you have to make that choice whether you think God is really speaking. Don't just do it because others have. Do it because God spoke to you.

God will always turn your sorrow into gladness and your pain into your testimony to help someone else. God promised me children long before I met my husband or had my first child. I received a word by a prophet of God about how many children I would have. I kept repeating the word I received back to God and now I see God's promises unfold before my eyes.

Sometimes people think that the road to your promise is going to be easy. Sometimes there may be a process before your promise, or obstacles you may have to endure. I can definitely say, I endured some obstacles, with each pregnancy, but God still hasn't forgotten his promise to me. About a year and a half ago, I received another word that I would conceive a girl. The bible says to believe his prophets. I believe that one day we will have a little girl.

The bible states in 2 Chronicles 20:20 And they rose early in the morning, and went forth into the wilderness of Tekoa: and as they went forth, Jehoshaphat stood and said, Hear me, O Judah, and ye inhabitants of Jerusalem; Believe in the LORD your

God, so shall ye be established; believe his prophets, so shall ye prosper.

Every time God speaks through Prophets of God concerning me and if it is a confirmation to my spirit, I believe. There are some of you that have been through multiple miscarriages, ectopic pregnancy, blighted ovum, still births etc. Any stage of loss is hard on a mother. Some people think that if a mother is only 6 weeks pregnant and she loses her child that it is not as significant as a mother who is 24 weeks. Although scientist will tell you their time line on when a fetus becomes a baby, to God there was a baby in your womb from day one of conception. Just as God has given me children He can bless you with children too.

Prayer over your womb:

Lord you have created me in your image and likeness. I speak to my womb now, and command it to come into alignment with the word of God. You said in your word ask and you shall receive, knock and the door will be open. I am believing for a child, and I know that you are a God of miracles. Heal every part of my body that would reject conception . God you said in Genesis to be fruitful and multiply. Lord your word is true and shall not turn back to me void. Just like Hannah, bless me with a child. Children are a heritage from the Lord. I believe in faith, and I Thank You that it is already done in the name of Jesus.

*There is such power in a husband that prays for his wife. Lay hands on your wife's stomach and declare wholeness and healing. Where two or three are gathered in his name there he is in the midst.

Chapter 6

SURPRISE

Boy was I surprised that I was pregnant for the fourth time. I paced the floor back and forth. We wanted our second son to be at least three, and I wanted to lose the weight from his pregnancy. We weren't using any birth control so I wasn't surprised that this happened. I have been writing this book since the beginning of this pregnancy, and everything that I wrote in the chapter "The Making of a King" is exactly what has happened during this pregnancy. I had a cerclage placed in at 15 weeks, and recovered for about a week. Currently I am 22 weeks, and I go back to the Doctor in about three weeks.

From week 18 to 20, I had something called Scatia. I have not been in so much pain in my whole life. The pain ran down from my back to my shin. I couldn't walk, get dressed or use the bathroom by myself. My husband would help me. The only pain reliever I could take was Tylenol, and that didn't help either. My Aunt that had some back pain recently told me to sit down for the most of the day. Prayer compiled with sitting down brought relief. After sitting for a week, and limiting my activities the pain was gone. It was a miracle. I couldn't imagine going through that for the rest of the pregnancy, let alone my husband going through it.

Originally we were not going to find out the gender, but we changed our mind. I asked the ultrasound tech to put the results in an envelope, so my husband and I could find out together that night. My husband opened that envelope, and said, "it's a boy". I thought that he was pulling my leg at first. I was surprised to find out we were having another boy. Earlier in the pregnancy, I had a dream that we had another boy, and that he looked like my youngest son.

Thus far, I have had lots of morning sickness, even past 12 weeks. I've had leg cramps, and some days I don't feel so great. I know that it will be all worth it at the end of this pregnancy. Don't give up on trying again. Keep trying until you get what God has promised you. Even though you may have lost your precious child, God will give you a miracle if you only believe. It is my prayer that you take hold to the word of God, just as Jacob said, "I will not let you go until you bless me". THERE IS NOTHING TOO HARD FOR GOD!

Chapter 7

DEALING WITH THE GRIEF

Grief is something most people will go through at least once in their lifetime. Grief is sorrow or distress over a particular person or thing. Grieving is a normal part of our human makeup. If you keep your emotions inside then you can make things worse. There is a period of time after the loss of a baby that you should grieve. Every body's time frame is different. The longer you hold on the more that grief can turn into sickness in your body.

Our bodies are only made to handle so much stress. It's called the "Fight or Flight" response. Once this hormone is activated, you can sometimes miss judge situations and not realize what is going on within you. Grief, if not dealt with can turn into depression, and other psychological disorders. You must decide to let go of that loved one. Yes, I know it's hard. Letting go can seem like you are trying to erase that person's memory from your mind, but in essence you are helping yourself. When you let go, you become whole. Healing does take time, and as time passes you will be stronger and stronger. Until one day you will have a memory and no longer respond the way you used to. If you are grieving and things are not getting better; go to a Christian counselor for help. A Christian counselor or Pastor can help you process what you have gone through according to scriptures. No one person will have all the answers, but there are resources that are available so you can get better.

Many times society tends to overlook the father in situations of miscarriage and loss. Yes, the mother has the closest bond to the baby, because she carried that child but, fathers also grieve the loss of their child. Sometimes after an event like this, family and friends call the mother, but the father doesn't receive any calls. Fathers are left to fend for themselves, as far as their feelings are concerned. As the man, he feels as if he needs to be strong for his wife. Men do cry. They may not cry in front of their wife, but they do release their emotions in some way or another. Some men may show their emotions in the form anger or isolation. It is important that we not forget about our other half, he may be grieving too.

I had one child when we lost our little girl. I did grieve as I mentioned in that chapter. It was two phone conversations with my mother and mother in law that helped me to realize what was in front of me. They said remember that you still have your son to take care of, he needs you. Sometimes if we are not careful, we can become so engulfed into the situation that we fail to realize the gifts in front of us. For me, emotions started to flood my mind about my first son being premature. Then now I had to deal with a loss. After a couple of months I finally felt like I was over it… and I was. I no longer cried over the thoughts of how she looked in that basket any more. You know, you may still cry years down the road every now and again, and that's because you are human. God has healed me from that loss and he can heal you too, if you put all your trust in Him.

Prayer for Grief:

Lord thank You that you bore all my pain on the cross. You feel this burden. I cast all my care upon You. Heal me where I hurt. Bring me through this trial. There is nothing too hard for You. Bottle up every tear and bring joy back into my life again. In Jesus name. Amen!

Chapter 8

EPILOGUE

Preemie Baby Prayer

God bless the little child behind the plastic wall. For all he knows is the ringing of the bells and the blurred images around him. He has been taken from my womb without warning and I long to hold him in my arms.

Lord, I ask in your name that my child be healed. I am willing to accept your decision no matter what it will be. I am willing to take on the responsibilities for caring for this child. I am willing to give this child love and understanding no matter the cost.

Please Lord help me to accept reality and what has happened without explanation or warning. Help me face the fact that this is not my fault and that I was given a special task to complete here on Earth.

God give my child the strength to make it through another second, minute, hour and day as each moment is a blessing and a triumph from heaven.

God, may you give the strength and compassion to the caregivers and nurses that take care of my child. May you keep my child protected and free from all injury and pain.

Please take away the guilt and burden from my heart dear Lord. It is heavy and I feel it is all my fault. Take it away dear Lord. Sweet Jesus allow me the strength and understanding I need to communicate with the Doctors and Nurses.

As you see dear Lord, I am at your mercy for the life of my child. Please leave him here on Earth and know that I will provide all the love and understanding that this child needs. I accept the challenge and will be your humble servant dear Lord.

~Author Unknown (http://project-angel-kisses.150m.com)

Miscarriage Poem

"Daddy please don't look so sad, momma please don't cry. Cause I'm in the arms of Jesus, and he sings me lullabies. Please try not to question God, don't think he is unkind. Don't think he sent me to you and then changed his mind. You see I'm a special child, I am needed up above. I'm the special gift you gave Him, a product of your love.

I'll always be there with you, so watch the sky at night. Look for the brightest star and know that's my halo's brilliant light. You'll see me in the morning frost that mists your window pane. That's me in the summer showers, I'll be dancing in the rain. When you feel a gentle breeze from a gentle wind that blows.

Know that it's me planting a kiss upon your nose. When you see a child playing and your heart feels a tug, Don't be sad mommy, that's just me giving your heart a hug. So daddy don't looks so sad and momma please don't cry. I'm in the arms of Jesus and he sings me lullabies!
~Author Unknown (grievingparents.com)

SCRIPTURES TO MEDITATE ON

Psalms 34:4
I sought the LORD, and he heard me, and delivered me from all my fears.

Psalms 34:18
The LORD is nigh unto them that are of a broken heart; and saveth such as be of a contrite spirit.

Psalms 55:22
Cast thy burden upon the LORD, and he shall sustain thee: he shall never suffer the righteous to be moved.

Proverbs 3:5,6
Trust in the LORD with all thine heart; and lean not unto thine own understanding. In all thy ways acknowledge him, and he shall direct thy paths.

Ecclesiaties 11:5
As thou knowest not what is the way of
the spirit, nor how the bones do grow in
the womb of her that is with child: even
so thou knowest not the works of God
who maketh all.

Isaiah 25:8
He will swallow up death in victory; and
the Lord GOD will wipe away tears from
off all faces; and the rebuke of his
people shall he take away from off all
the earth: for the LORD hath spoken it.

Isaiah 40:29-31
He giveth power to the faint; and to
them that have no might he increaseth
strength. Even the youths shall faint
and be weary, and the young men shall
utterly fall: But they that wait upon
the LORD shall renew their strength;
they shall mount up with wings as
eagles; they shall run, and not be weary;
and they shall walk, and not faint.

Isaiah 41:10

Fear thou not; for I am with thee: be not dismayed; for I am thy God: I will strengthen thee; yea, I will help thee; yea, I will uphold thee with the right hand of my righteousness.

Matthew 11:28-30

Come unto me, all ye that labour and are heavy laden, and I will give you rest. Take my yoke upon you, and learn of me; for I am meek and lowly in heart: and ye shall find rest unto your souls. For my yoke is easy, and my burden is light.

Romans 8:28

And we know that all things work together for good to them that love God, to them who are the called according to his purpose.

Philippians 4:4-7

Rejoice in the Lord always: and again I say, Rejoice. Let your moderation be known unto all men. The Lord is at hand. Be careful for nothing; but in everything by prayer and supplication with thanksgiving let your requests be made known unto God. And the peace of God, which passeth all understanding, shall keep your hearts and minds through Christ Jesus.

Hebrews 10:36

For ye have need of patience, that, after ye have done the will of God, ye might receive the promise.

ABOUT THE AUTHOR

Author Krystle Lynch is the wife of Gabriel and Stay at home mom to two beautiful children; and one on the way. It is her goal to reach any woman that has suffered from miscarriage, preterm birth and loss. God has turned her mourning into dancing. She is a servant in Gods kingdom and is called to reach hurting women.

www.ingramcontent.com/pod-product-compliance
Lightning Source LLC
Chambersburg PA
CBHW072343290526
45794CB00002B/996